DR BARBARA NATURAL TREATMENT FOR ERECTILE DYSFUNCTION

The Complete Guide to Alkaline Herbal Cure for Erectile Dysfunction Using Dr Barbara O'Neill Diet

Kathona Bodi

ISBN: 9798333282316

CONTENTS

Introduction

Erectile dysfunction (ED) is something that many men experience at one point in their lives or another. In fact, it is reported that over 50 percent of men between 40 and 70 years old deal with some form of ED. So, it's comforting to know that you are not in the struggle alone.

Not being able to get an erection or maintain it from time to time can happen for various reasons. For most men, this usually occurs after consuming a lot of alcohol or going through periods of stress.

While there is no magic supplement or food that can prevent ED or resolve the problem, studies show that your diet and a combination of other lifestyle factors can go a long way in helping you deal with the problem. In general, a healthy diet may help to maintain erectile function, enabling you to have firmer and more reliable erections. I'm talking about foods like vegetables, whole grains and fruits. On the other hand, foods such as fried foods, red meat and alcohol can contribute to ED and other health problems.

This book focuses on treating erectile dysfunction through a plant-based approach. Specifically, we will be following the Dr Barbara diet which essentially consists of alkaline formulations that can help deal with ED. Barbara is a famous nutritionist who advocates for alternative medicine. She's a strong believer in the power of food to cure various diseases including ED.

What Is Erectile Dysfunction?

Let's start by answering an important question - what is erectile dysfunction?

Erectile dysfunction is simply when a male has trouble getting or maintaining an erection. This can happen at least 20 percent of the time, where the penis does not get hard enough or it gets hard but softens too soon.

While this can be embarrassing, especially if you need to talk about it, it is important to know that the condition is quite common. In fact, over 30 million males in the US have experienced this problem.

Having an erectile problem can affect your quality of life and may lead to problems in your relationship. In some cases, it can lead to anxiety, which may cause you to lose self-esteem.

What Causes Erectile Dysfunction?

So, what actually causes ED? Well, it can be linked to various reasons. Sometimes, it may occur as a side effect of a particular drug or medication. It can also be caused by stress, which might come from your job or relationship, as well as depression.

For more than 70 percent of men, the cause can be a bit more complex. The condition may arise due to an underlying health condition, surgery, or prostate treatment. Examples of such conditions include diabetes, vascular problems, and neurological disease.

In many cases, the major contributor to erectile dysfunction are clogged arteries which cause insufficient supply of blood to the penis. In other words, it's actually a cardiovascular problem leading up to ED.

In general, the causes of erectile dysfunction can be said to be either physical or psychological (emotional).

Examples of physical causes include:

- Insufficient blood supply (a situation often attributed to atherosclerosis, which is the hardening of the arteries)
- Nervous system problems (usually a deficit in nerve signaling which can be caused by a spinal cord injury or brain injury)
- Hormonal issues
- Medications
- Smoking too much and the use of alcohol
- Pelvis surgery or injury
- Etc.

Men with underlying health conditions such as cardiovascular disease, obesity, high cholesterol, and diabetes are usually at greater risk of developing ED.

The emotional side of things which can also contribute to the condition includes anxiety, depression, and stress.

Does Diet Have An Impact On Erectile Dysfunction?

There's no better way to approach a problem, especially when it has to do with the body than to look at the root cause.

For erectile dysfunction, more often, there's an underlying health problem responsible, which could be diabetes, high cholesterol level, diabetes, or a cardiovascular condition. Interestingly, when treating these diseases, the first line of action often involves making changes to one's diet and exercise.

So, while there are several factors and lifestyles that can contribute to ED, studies have shown that there's often a direct link between diet and erectile dysfunction.

That is why one of the best ways to prevent ED is to adhere to a healthy diet. This is why the Dr Barbara diet works so well because it's plant-based and focuses on eliminating all the bad stuff.

Why the Dr Barbara Alkaline Diet Works

When it comes to preventing or managing erectile dysfunction, a Mediterranean diet is often recommended. While this does work, I have realized that it's often better to fully go plant-based. This is because a Mediterranean diet essentially consists of consuming plant-based foods but replaces meat with fish.

However, there are many plant-based sources of Omega 3 for vegans which seems healthier. These include nuts and seeds such as chia seeds, flaxseed, and walnuts, as well as plant oils like canola, soybean oil, and olive oil.

The Dr Barbara Diet is fully plant-based and consists of eating fresh veggies, fruits, whole grains, and Omega 3 rich foods like nuts and seeds.

Studies have shown people who eat more fresh plant-based foods such as fruits are 14 percent less likely to experience erectile dysfunction than those who eat very little. While the Dr Barbara diet focuses on limiting your consumption of processed foods, I would say it's better you completely eliminate it from your diet when dealing with ED.

But it shouldn't end with your diet, there's also a need to increase your physical activity if you are serious about making progress.

In general, whether you want to prevent ED or treat it, you will need to combine a plant-based diet (Dr Barbara) and increase your physical activity (exercise). If you need to use dietary supplements, make sure you do so in moderation.

Why Physical Activity is Important

Exercise and physical activity is not only important for ED but also help to improve your overall health. Some of the benefits include:

- Reducing your risk for diabetes
- Improving your cardiovascular health
- Reducing or maintaining your weight
- Improving brain health
- Improving cardiovascular health
- Preventing or managing cardiovascular diseases
- Reducing symptoms of anxiety and depression
- Reducing high blood sugar

As you may have already discovered, I'm not a big fan of taking pills for ED because I believe they only treat the symptoms and provide a temporary solution.

For long-term results, there needs to be a complete overhaul of one's diet and lifestyle. A plant-based way of eating will not only increase your longevity but also aid your metabolic health. Believe me, I'm talking from experience.

While I don't advocate a total ban on meat, I believe it's best if you fully adopt a plant-rich lifestyle as prescribed by Dr Barbara. Even if you need to eat meat, it has to be in the least amount and you have to be mindful of the type of meat. Personally, I would rather you have fish, especially healthy sources of Omega-3 fats such as salmon, sardines, and trout.

Fasting and Erectile Dysfunction

Another thing you can do to improve your erectile function is fasting. Not many people know this, but intermittent fasting, or fasting generally, can help men rise to the occasion and decrease the risk of various chronic health conditions including type 2 diabetes.

This is usually the case when you combine intermittent fasting and an organic diet. In fact, people who do these two are less likely to develop ED. But even for people who already have this condition, switching to an organic diet accompanied by intermittent fasting can be a game changer.

Before we go on, let's start with the basics for people who are new to intermittent fasting.

What Is Intermittent Fasting?

We already know that fasting means to go without food for a specific period of time.

Intermittent fasting is simply when you alternate between periods of eating and fasting according to a strict, routine schedule. A practical example is what Muslims do during Ramadan. During this period, Muslims keep a daily fast, which usually lasts from dawn to sunset. So, they go for 14 hours daily without eating or drinking.

Studies show that fasting for a couple of hours daily offers a lot of health benefits including reducing fat and controlling type 2 diabetes, which are known risk factors for ED.

So, how does obesity and diabetes increase your risk of having ER?

Well, whenever a man gets "in the mood", a certain chemical compound called nitric oxide is released, which sends a signal that tells the muscles and arteries to relax and allow more blood flow to the penis. This is what causes you to have an erection.

Unfortunately, when your blood sugar level is too high, it reduces the amount of nitric oxide that is released, which results in insufficient blood flow that is required to start and maintain a strong erection.

Besides high blood sugar which causes poor blood supply, diabetes is another condition that can affect a man's erectile function. When a man is overweight, it reduces the amount of testosterone they can produce. Also, testosterone is converted to oestrogen (a female hormone) by fat cells, which reduces the male libido and results in a weaker erection.

How Fasting Can Help With Erectile Dysfunction

In order to fully understand how fasting can help with ER, let's first understand how it can be used to prevent diabetes.

Fasting and Diabetes Prevention

When you go on an intermittent fast, what happens is that your blood glucose level becomes elevated when you eat but remains for the rest of the day. This means that, if you fast for at least 6-8 hours, the glucose from your last meals will become exhausted, then the body will begin to look for other sources of fuel.

At this point, a process kicks in, known as glucogenesis, where glucose is made from stored fats or proteins. Consequently, this brings down the blood sugar while reducing fat and increasing insulin sensitivity. This is how fasting can help protect against diabetes.

Since fasting reduces blood sugar, this means it can increase the production of nitric oxide since higher blood sugar reduces the release of nitric oxide.

This allows for optimal blood flow required to start and maintain a strong erection.

In addition, fasting reduces body fat, which increases the level of male hormones and reduces fat in the belly region.

As a result, men who fast will have a healthier sex drive than men who don't. A lower belly fat will also result in a longer-looking penis.

Studies have repeatedly shown that combining intermittent fasting with a vegan diet is more effective for preventing or treating ER than just following a vegan diet alone.

So, even though I'm an advocate of a plant-based diet such as Dr Barbara's, you will achieve better results when you combine it with fasting.

That is why I have spent so much time talking about fasting.

How to Get Started With Intermittent Fasting

There are two common ways to approach intermittent fasting. You can either have a time-restricted eating daily or practice the 5:2 diet.

Let's go over each one in detail.

Daily time-restricted eating

When doing a time-restricted eating fast, you can only eat within a specific time window. In other words, you will have periods of eating and fasting each day. This can go on for many days - 10, 14, 21, 40 or even 100 days. Some people may even fast this way for up to 6 months.

In terms of how long, there are many variants but the more common ones are a 16-hour fast and 8-hour eating window, 18-hour fast and 6-hour eating window, and 20-hour fast and 4-hour eating window. Usually, the longer you fast, the better for you as your body will be more sensitive to insulin.

During your eating window, I highly recommend you don't eat more than twice.

For instance, if you're doing a 16-hour fast and 8-hour eating window, during the 8-hour window, try not to eat more than twice and avoid the temptation to overeat just to make up for the times you're not eating. So, eat your normal portion or less and drink a lot of water, especially during the times you're not eating.

You may also choose to eat just once throughout the whole day instead of twice. This type of fasting is known as OMAD (one meal a day) and happens to be my favorite.

The 5:2 diet

With the 5:2 diet, you eat normally for the first 5 days in a week (or out of a 7-day period). For the remaining 2 days, either you completely abstain from food or you eat a very small amount (usually not more than 300-400 calories).

If the idea of going 16 hours without food or eating only 300 calories twice per week sounds too restrictive, you can take alkaline juices or smoothies during the periods of fasting to help stave off hunger. Zero-calorie beverages are also allowed.

What Other Things Can Help To Improve Your Libido?

Like I said earlier, you should engage in a lot of physical activities. Specifically, one of the best exercises for improving erectile function is kegel.

While kegel exercises are quite common among women, they can also be very useful to men struggling with ED.

This is because it helps to strengthen the bulbocavernosus muscle that surrounds the base of the penis, which helps to control erection and ejaculation.

When performing kegel exercise, try to activate the muscles that stop urination midstream and hold for at least 6 seconds, then relax. You should repeat this 10-20 times, 2-3 times a day.

Another exercise you can do is walking. Studies show that walking just 30 minutes a day can decrease ED by up to 41 percent.

Overall, you should plan to exercise at least 4 days per week, and it doesn't have to be anything intense; just moderate exercise is enough.

In addition to exercise, you want to avoid other unhealthy lifestyles such as smoking and alcohol consumption.

Coffee can also help as it's loaded with antioxidants. Thanks to its caffeine content, it can also help to boost blood flow and relax the arteries. Studies have shown that drinking two to three cups of coffee daily reduces the risk of ED.

Counseling may also help, especially if you've gotten to the point where ED has become an emotional issue. Talking to someone, especially an expert, may help to clear up your

mind while you're working towards recovery.

Best Foods for Erectile Dysfunction

Now let's look at some of the best alkaline-forming foods for erectile dysfunction based on the Dr Barbara diet.

Generally, the best diet for erectile function is one rich in fruits, whole grains, and vegetables. This is why the Dr Barbara diet works so well. However, let's look at individual foods that seem to offer the most benefit for ER.

- Flavonoid-rich fruits such as blackberries
- Watermelon (contains L-citrulline which helps to stimulate blood flow)
- Dark leafy greens such as spinach, asparagus, and Brussels sprouts
- Oatmeal (also contains L-arginine which is known to increase blood flow)
- Almonds, hazelnuts, walnuts, and pistachios

- Avocados (contain high levels of zinc which may increase testosterone production)
- Pomegranate juice
- Bananas (rich in potassium and flavonoids, which reduces the risk of ED)
- Foods rich in Omega-3 fatty acids such as edamame, walnuts, chia seeds, flaxseed, etc.
- Chili pepper (may help stimulate the circulatory system, which can affect your blood vessels and increase blood flow)
- Peanuts (also rich in arginine which can help boost nitric oxide levels)
- Coffee and dark chocolate
- Cocoa (also rich in flavonoids)
- Whole grains
- Herbs and spices
- Olive oil
- Garlic

Worst Foods for Erectile Dysfunction

- Alcohol

- Sugary drinks

- Soy-based products

- Licorice

- Fried foods (such as French fries, egg rolls, fried chicken, mozzarella strips, corn dogs, etc.)

- Red meat (e.g. beef, mutton, pork, lamb, etc.)

- Foods high in sodium such as tacos, burgers, seafood, pizza, and so on

- Processed foods

- Junks

- Tobacco (smoking)

Dr Barbara Alkaline Recipes for Erectile Dysfunction

KALE SALAD & HEMP RANCH

Ingredients

- One teaspoon of dill
- Half a teaspoon of sea salt
- Half a cup of hemp seeds
- Two tablespoons of squeezed lime juice
- Half butternut squash, cubed
- Six cups of chopped kale
- Two teaspoons of salt
- One to two tablespoons of grapeseed oil

Instructions

1. Switch on the oven and heat it to up to 350-400 degrees F.

2. Put the hemp seeds, dill, and lime juice in a blender and blend until smooth. You can also use a food processor.

3. Now, toss the kale and squash in the grapeseed oil and add the sea salt. Transfer to a baking dish and roast for 15 to 20 minutes or until cooked. You will know this when the kale gets crispy.

4. Allow to cook, then you can top with dressings.

AVOCADO LETTUCE WRAPS

Ingredients

- One teaspoon of sea salt
- Two avocados, sliced
- One teaspoon of fresh lime juice
- Twelve romaine lettuce leaves
- Two diced bell peppers
- Half red onion (should be diced and sliced)
- Three plum tomatoes, chopped
- One to two teaspoons of cayenne pepper

Instructions

1. Mix all the ingredients in a bowl except the romaine lettuce.
2. Next, you want to wash the lettuce separately. Allow it to dry.
3. Now, place the dry leaves on a plate or dish in such a way that each one forms a natural scoop.
4. Next, pour the mixture you prepared from step one into each leaf so that it fills it. Now, you have your avocado lettuce wraps. Enjoy!

RYE TOMATO & AVOCADO SANDWICH

Ingredients

- Two slices of rye bread
- Two sliced plum tomatoes
- One avocado, sliced
- One to two teaspoons of sea salt
- One to three tablespoons of olive oil
- Half a cup of dandelion greens or purslane

Instructions

1. Place the avocado slices on top of the bread slices.
2. Next, drizzle with olive oil. It should go on top of the avocado.
3. Now, arrange the tomato slices on top of the avocados. You can sprinkle some salt if you wish.
4. Finally, top with purslane. Enjoy your sandwich.

ELECTRIC SALAD

Ingredients

- 1 cup cherry tomatoes
- 2 red onions
- 1 handful romaine lettuce
- 1 lime (you will need the juice)
- 1 cup kale, chopped
- 3 jalapenos
- Olive oil

- 1 yellow pepper
- 1 orange pepper

Instructions

1. The first thing is to wash and rinse all the ingredients if you have not already done so. Once dry, cut them into smaller pieces.
2. Combine everything in a bowl and drizzle with the lemon juice and oil. Enjoy!

QUINOA PORRIDGE

Ingredients

- ½ tsp cayenne
- ½ lime (you will need to grate the skin)
- 1 cup dry quinoa
- 2 cups water

- ½ cup coconut milk (can be substituted with cream if you wish)
- Cloves to taste
- ½ handful assorted nuts and seeds (optional)

Instructions

1. Prepare the quinoa according to the instructions on the package.
2. After that, pour it into a saucepan (this should be after you have drained the quinoa). Then add the cloves and cayenne. Stir well to combine.
3. Next, add the milk and grated lime (you can also add grated apple if you wish). Stir well to mix.
4. Top with nuts and seeds. Enjoy!

ALKALINE MILLET

Ingredients

- ½ tsp sea salt
- 2 ½ cup water
- 1 cup millet

Instructions

1. The first thing is to dry sauté the millet until golden brown. Then add in the water and salt.
2. Bring the mixture to a boil, then simmer until the water is absorbed. This usually takes about 30 minutes but it could be more depending on the heat.
3. Let everything cool with the lid on. Serve and enjoy!

ZUCCHINI AND HEART MUSHROOM SOUP

Ingredients

- 1 medium zucchini, chopped
- 1 medium-sized onion, chopped (if you eat onion a lot, then you can use a large onion instead)
- 2 bay leaves

- Any vegetable stock of your choice (ideally, homemade)
- 1 tsp grapeseed oil
- 1 lb mushroom, mixed and chopped
- Cayenne pepper to taste
- Sea salt to taste
- Sweet basil to taste

Instructions

1. Start by setting your stove to medium heat. Set a pan with a heavy base on top of the stove, then add the grapeseed oil. Once it gets a little hot, add in the onion and sauté for 5 minutes.
2. Next, add the mushrooms, basil, and bay leaves. Allow it to cook for an additional five minutes, then add the zucchini. Cook until the vegetables release their juices. This might take up to 10-15 minutes.
3. Now, pour in the vegetable stock and bring to a boil. Then reduce the heat and simmer for five minutes.
4. Finally, remove the bay leaves from the soup before seasoning with salt and pepper. Serve!

MUSHROOM & ONION GRAVY

Ingredients

- 2-3 cups of spring water
- ½ cup mushroom
- 1 tsp sea salt
- ½ cup onion
- ½ tsp oregano
- ¼ cup cayenne
- ½ tsp thyme
- 2 tbsp grapeseed oil
- 3 tbsp garbanzo bean flour
- 1 tsp onion powder

Instructions

1. Start by pouring the grapeseed oil into your frying pan. Then set it on the stove over medium or high heat.

2. Once the oil is a bit hot, add the onion and mushroom and sauté for a minute. Then add the other seasonings and spices, except the cayenne.

3. Sauté for five minutes, then add 2 cups of spring water and the cayenne. Stir well to mix and allow to boil.

4. While you're waiting, sift in the flour little by little, then use a whisk to stir it well in order to reduce lumps.

5. Continue cooking until it boils. You can add more water if you want but don't add not more than one cup. Serve.

GINGER TEA

Ingredients

- 1 pinch cayenne
- 1 thumb fresh ginger root (can be substituted with the powder)
- 4 cups spring water

- 2 tbsp fresh lime juice

- 2 sprigs of new organic dill weed

- Raw agave to taste

Instructions

1. Start by boiling the spring water.

2. While you're waiting, peel the ginger root, then chop it into tiny pieces and add to the boiling water. Also, add the weed.

3. Let it cook for 5 minutes, then strain the tea into a glass jar. Add the lime juice and cayenne and stir.

4. Finally, add the agave to taste. You can have it either hot or cold.

AVOCADO BOWL

Ingredients

- Fresh lime juice from 1 lime

- ½ cup cucumber, chopped

- 2 tbsp melted coconut oil
- 16-20 basil leaves (can be substituted with parsley leaves)
- 1 avocado
- Nuts, chopped
- ⅛ tsp lime zest (you can use more for serving)
- 1 pinch salt
- Agave to taste (optional)

Instructions

1. Start by pouring the lime juice into a blender. Add the avocado and agave. Then blend the mixture until smooth.
2. Now, add the lime zest, cucumber, salt, and coconut oil. Blend again until smooth.
3. Then add the basil or parsley leaves and mix a bit.
4. Transfer to a bowl and top with the chopped nuts. You can top with more lime zest if desired.

FRUIT SALAD

Ingredients

- One pint of fresh blueberries
- One ripe pear, cored and diced
- One pint of fresh strawberries, sliced (no stems)
- Two cups grapes, deseeded
- 2 tbsp date syrup (optional)
- ¼ tsp ground cinnamon
- 2 tbsp freshly squeezed lemon juice

Instructions

1. Combine all the ingredients in a bowl. Store in a refrigerator. Serve chill.

HERBERT HUMMUS

Ingredients

- Two garlic cloves
- One cup of fresh basil leaves, blanched and lightly packed
- Four cups of cooked garbanzo beans
- Juice from one lemon
- One cup of vegetable broth
- Half a cup of tarragon leaves, blanched and lightly packed
- Half a cup of fresh, flat parsley leaves
- ¼ cup of chives, chopped
- 2 tbsp sesame seeds, toasted

Instructions

1. Start by dabbing the basil leaves and tarragon until they dry. Now, cut them into smaller bits and put in a blender or food processor.
2. Add in the beans, sesame seeds, lemon juice, garlic, and vegetable broth. Blend until smooth and creamy. Add the chives; stir and serve.

NB: Consume within 4 days.

MISO NOODLE SOUP

Ingredients

- Two scallions, sliced
- One cup of adzuki beans (cooked or canned)
- Four tablespoons of miso
- Two tablespoons of fresh cilantro/basil, chopped
- Seven ounces of soba noodles (100% buckwheat)
- Four cups of water

Instructions

1. Start by pouring some water into a large pot; bring it to a boil.
2. Next, add in the soba noodles and stir. Cook for about five minutes, then drain and rinse (use hot water).

3. In another pot, pour in some water and bring to boil. Remove from heat and add in the miso and stir until dissolved.

4. Finally, add the noodles, adzuki beans, scallions and cilantro to the miso broth. Stir well to combine. Serve warm.

HEMP MILK

Ingredients

- Spring water
- 6 tbsp sea moss gel
- 1 cup hemp seeds

Instructions

1. Start by soaking the hemp seeds in 6 cups of spring water for 30 minutes.

2. Next, transfer the seeds with the water into a blender and blend until smooth.

3. Add in the sea moss and blend for 30 seconds. Store in the refrigerator and use within four days.

TASTY PANINI

Ingredients

- 1 tsp cinnamon
- ¼ cup natural peanut butter
- ¼ cup raisin
- ¼ cup hot water
- Whole grain bread, 2 slices
- 1 ripe banana, peeled and chopped
- 2 tsp cacao powder

Instructions

1. Start by pouring the hot water into a bowl. Add the cinnamon, raisin, and cacao powder and combine.
2. Next, spread the peanut butter on each of the bread slices.

3. Place the chopped banana on the toast.

4. Next, transfer the raisin mixture into a blender and
    blend until smooth. Spread on the sandwich. Enjoy!

BASIC POLENTA

Ingredients

- One and a half cups of coarse cornmeal
- Five cups of water
- ¾ tsp salt

Instructions

1. Start by pouring the water into a saucepan. Put it on
    a stove and set to low heat.

2. Gradually add the cornmeal into the water. Then stir
    until creamy. This might take a couple of minutes.

3. Season with the salt, then transfer the polenta into a
    bowl. Refrigerate for an hour, then serve.

PECANS & BERRIES SALAD

Ingredients

- Baby arugula or mixed baby greens (15 oz pack)

- Blackberries (half pack, should weigh up to 3 oz)

- Raspberries (half pack, should weigh up to 3 oz)

- Fifteen pecan halves

To make the vinaigrette, here's what you need:

- 3 tbsp extra virgin olive oil

- $\frac{1}{8}$ tsp kosher salt

- $\frac{1}{8}$ tsp freshly ground pepper to taste

- 1 tbsp champagne vinegar (or rice vinegar/ apple cider vinegar)

- $\frac{1}{2}$ tsp dried basil

Instructions

1. Let's start with the dressing/vinaigrette. Pour the vinegar into a bowl (make sure it's a bowl that won't react with the vinegar). Now add in the basil, pepper, and salt.

2. Next, you want to emulsify the olive oil with the vinaigrette. To do this, drizzle the oil in a slow stream; then whisk together until emulsified.

3. Now, combine the vinaigrette and baby arugula (or mixed greens) and transfer to a salad bowl.

4. Top with pecans, raspberries, and blackberries. Serve immediately.

BUTTERNUT SQUASH SOUP

Ingredients

- One tablespoon of olive oil
- One small onion, chopped
- Two tablespoons of fresh sage, chopped

- Six cups of butternut squash (peeled and cubed, should weigh about 30 oz)
- Half a teaspoon of kosher salt or sea salt
- One sweet apple (ideally, it should be large in size, you will need to peel and chop it)
- Half a teaspoon of cinnamon, grounded
- Half a teaspoon of paprika
- Four and a half cups of vegetable broth
- One tablespoon of fresh ginger, grated
- Half a cup of coconut milk (you can use more for garnish)
- ¼ tsp fresh nutmeg, grated

Instructions

1. Start by preheating your oven to 400 degrees F. Next, mix the apple, sage, squash, cinnamon, onion, paprika, and ¼ tsp salt in a Dutch oven. Toss in one tablespoon of olive oil and combine very well.
2. Roast until the squash becomes tender. This usually takes about half an hour.

3. After that, transfer the Dutch oven to the stove and add in the coconut milk, broth, nutmeg, ginger, and ¼ tsp salt. Allow to boil.

4. Next, you want to blend the mixture. You can either use an immersion blender or you can transfer the soup to the blender in batches. Blend until you get a smooth consistency.

5. When serving, you can drizzle extra coconut milk on top and if you like, add a pinch of nutmeg.

CARROT BANANA PROTEIN DRINK

Ingredients

- ¼ cup unflavored pea protein powder (you can substitute this with whey protein)
- Half a teaspoon of turmeric
- One cup of almond milk
- One medium-sized banana, riped
- Two baby carrots
- One tablespoon of ground flax

- Agave syrup (or any other natural sweetener of your choice)
- Ice

Instructions

1. Add all the ingredients to a blender and blend until you get a smooth consistency. Enjoy!

SUPERFOOD SMOOTHIE

Ingredients

- 1 date, pitted
- Half medium-sized banana, riped
- Half a tablespoon of chia seeds
- One tablespoon of raw shelled hemp seeds (you can substitute this with any other seed of your choice)
- ¾ cup of baby kale or spinach
- ¾ cup unsweetened vanilla almond milk

- One cup of ice

Instructions

1. Add everything to a blender or high-speed food processor and blend until you get a smooth consistency. Enjoy!

LEMON BRUSSEL SPROUTS

Ingredients

- ¼ cup fresh lemon juice
- Half a cup of chicken broth or low-sodium vegetable broth
- Zest from one lemon
- Two pounds of Brussel sprouts, the ends should be trimmed
- Two teaspoons of kosher salt
- ¼ teaspoon of fresh ground pepper

Instructions

1. Start by shredding the sprouts; you can do this with the slicing disk on a food processor or a sharp knife. If you're using a sharp knife, you will need to halve the sprouts before thinly slicing by hand.
2. Pour the broth into a deep skillet and heat over medium heat. Once it begins to simmer, add in the shredded sprouts and season with the pepper and salt.
3. Sauté and stir frequently until the sprouts become a little wilted. This should take about 8-10 minutes. Then remove the skillet from heat.
4. You can stir in the lemon zest and juice if you plan to serve right away, otherwise stir in the lemon just before you serve it hot or warm anytime.

CHOCOLATE BANANA DRINK

Ingredients

- Six ounces of carob-flavored soy milk (can be substituted with fortified cocoa)
- One banana, diced and frozen
- One pinch of cinnamon

Instructions

1. Combine everything in a blender and blend until smooth. Serve immediately.

KIWIFRUIT SHAKE

Ingredients

- 4 cups non-fat vanilla vegan yogurt, frozen
- 2 sliced kiwifruit

Instructions

1. Add both ingredients to a blender or food processor
   and blend until smooth. Serve.

LEMON QUINOA SALAD

Ingredients

- One cup of lentils, cooked
- One cup of quinoa, cooked
- Three tablespoons of olive oil
- One minced garlic clove
- Half a cup of yellow bell pepper, chopped
- Half a cup of red bell pepper, chopped
- ¼ cup freshly squeezed lemon juice
- ¼ cup red onion, chopped
- Salt to taste

Instructions

1. Combine all the ingredients (except salt) in a large bowl. Season with salt to taste.

2. You can season with more grounded pepper if you wish. Serve.

GRANOLA PLATE

Things You Need

- Two and a half cups of oats
- A cup of shredded coconut, unsweetened without preservatives
- 1 tsp of vanilla, extract
- ¾ cup of almonds
- ¼ cup of maple syrup (should be pure)
- ¼ cup of pumpkin seeds
- ½ cup of walnuts (only use if you tolerate it)
- ¼ tsp cinnamon (optional)

- ⅛ tsp of sea salt

- 2 tbsp of coconut oil

- Dried mango to taste (optional, must come without any preservatives)

Cooking Instructions

1. Start by preheating your oven. Set the temperature at 300 degrees Fahrenheit.

2. Transfer the almonds, oats, and walnuts onto cookie sheet.

3. Next, get a small pot and mix the other ingredients - coconut oil, syrup, cinnamon, salt and vanilla. Now pour the mixture on top of the oats and walnuts and flip to mix it up.

4. Then bake for 18-22 minutes. Make sure to stir every 8-10 minutes.

5. When you're done, take it out of the oven, then add the pumpkin seeds and coconut.

6. Bake for an extra 10 to 15 minutes, then take it out and move to a Pyrex dish to get it to cool. Once again, you want to stir often.

7. Optionally, you can cut the dried mango into tiny slices and mix with the granola. Otherwise, skip this step if it's not tolerated. Put it in the fridge to cool.

"MINT" ICED TEA

Things You Need

- 1 tbsp of mint leaves (fresh, ideally should come in a sachet or tea ball)
- Chamomile tea (a bag should be enough)
- 1 teaspoon of sweetener (agave syrup/you can also use raw honey though this is not permitted in Dr Barbara's guide)

Cooking Instructions

1. Get a medium-sized teapot and fill it with water. Now, soak (or steep) the tea for 18-20 minutes.

2. Remove the mint and chamomile. Add your preferred sweetener and stir well. Allow it to cool down, then put it in the fridge.

WATERMELON SALAD

Things You Need

- One red watermelon (small or half-size, seedless)
- One to two cups of English cucumber (sliced)
- Mint sprigs to taste (make sure it's fresh)
- ***Blueberries (one half-pint box)***

Cooking Instructions

1. Slice the watermelon into tiny pieces. Next, "scrape off" the outer part, then cut into very small chunks.
2. Transfer the chunks to 1 large bowl or you can divide it into smaller bowls.
3. Next, add the cucumber slices and use the blueberries and sprigs as toppings.

Sweet Potato & Peanut Curry

Ingredients

- A piece of thumb-sized ginger, grated
- 200g bag of spinach
- One tablespoon of coconut oil
- Two cloves of garlic, grated
- One onion, chopped
- One lime, juiced
- 400ml can of coconut milk
- Three tablespoons of Thai red curry paste (ensure it's vegan, you can check for this on the label or packaging)
- One tablespoon of peanut butter
- 500g of sweet potato (after peeling, cut it into small chunks)
- Water

Instructions

1. Start by melting the coconut oil in a saucepan over medium heat. Then add the onion and saute for 4-5 minutes.
2. Next, add in the garlic cloves and ginger and cook for another one minute until the fragrance is released.
3. Now, stir in the other ingredients - curry paste, peanut butter, coconut milk, and sweet potato. Add in about 200 ml of water.
4. Allow the mixture to boil, then reduce the heat and simmer for an additional 20 minutes or until the potatoes become soft. The cover of the saucepan should be removed during this period.
5. Finally, stir in the spinach and lime juice and add your favorite seasoning. Serve alone or with cooked rice (ideally, brown rice or whole grain rice)

Mango & Avocado Salsa

Ingredients

- One garlic clove, minced
- Two tablespoons of fresh lime juice
- One ripe mango (make sure to peel and dice it before use)
- One jalapeno, seeded and diced
- One plum tomato, diced
- One medium Hass avocado, diced
- Half a tablespoon of olive oil
- Two tablespoons of fresh lime juice
- ¼ cup fresh cilantro, chopped
- ¼ cup red onion, chopped
- Pepper and kosher salt to taste

Instructions

1. Mix all the ingredients together in a bowl. Then put it in a refrigerator to marinate for about 30 minutes. Enjoy.

Zucchini & Plum Tomatoes

Ingredients

- Half a tablespoon of Herbes de Provence (you can find how to make this online)
- One medium-sized zucchini (cut into bits)
- Five medium-sized fresh plum tomatoes, diced
- Two tablespoons of extra virgin olive oil
- Five garlic cloves, smashed
- Fresh pepper and kosher salt to taste

Instructions

1. Pour the olive oil into a large non-stick skillet and heat. Set the stove to medium-high heat.
2. Add in the garlic and sauté until it turns golden. This should take about a minute or two.
3. Now, add in salt and pepper followed by zucchini.

4. Leave it to cook for 4 to 5 minutes on each side. Then introduce the plum tomatoes and Herbes de Provence. You can add additional salt if you desire.

5. Reduce the heat and simmer for 5 to 10 minutes. Serve.

Baked Bananas

Ingredients

- 1 banana (ideally, it should be medium ripped; cut it into half lengthwise)
- Half a tablespoon of honey
- Cinnamon to taste

Instructions

1. Start by preheating the oven to 400 degrees F.

2. Arrange the banana halves on a foil or oven-safe dish. Sprinkle with honey and cinnamon.

3. Cover tight with foil, then place it in the oven and allow to bake for 10-15 minutes. Enjoy!

4. Optionally, you can serve with light ice cream or whipped cream.

Butternut Squash Lentil Soup

Ingredients

- One bay leaf
- One large onion, diced
- One celery stalk, diced
- One medium-sized carrot, diced
- Half a tablespoon of olive oil
- Six cups of vegetable broth
- Two leeks (we will need only the white part; clean and chop into smaller pieces)
- Two tablespoons of tomato paste

- One pound of butternut, peeled and diced into half inches
- Two ounces of green lentils (this is equivalent to ⅓ cup)
- Three cups of packed chopped lacinato kale (the stems should be removed)
- Half a teaspoon of kosher salt

Instructions

1. Start by heating a Dutch oven or some other heavy pot over medium heat.
2. Once it gets hot, add the olive oil, and follow up with the onions, celery, leeks, and carrots. Reduce the heat and let it cook for 4-5 minutes as you stir it.
3. Now, add in the tomato paste and let it cook for an additional two minutes while stirring.
4. Pour in the vegetable broth, lentils, and bay leaf and allow to boil. Then reduce the heat, cover the pot and simmer for about 20 minutes.
5. Introduce the butternut and cook until tender. This should take up to 15 minutes or more.

6. Remove the bay leaf, then add salt and pepper as
   seasoning. Now, add in the kale and allow to cook
   for 5 to 7 minutes or until the kale becomes tender.

Conclusion

I would like to end it here. I hope you found the information in this book helpful in your journey to overcome erectile dysfunction.

The truth is that sex can be seen as a sport. As a middle-aged man, you may not be able to run as fast as you did in your 20s or hit a baseball as far as you usually do. But even with this natural decline that comes with aging, it doesn't mean you should go out of league. There are still plenty of ways to stay in the game and enjoy your sex life. That is what a healthier lifestyle can do for you.

I hope you put into practice everything you've learned in this book, especially when it comes to eliminating the bad stuff and following the Dr. Barbara diet. I hope to hear your testimonies soon.